NATURAL URINARY TRACT INFECTION (UTI) TREATMENT

DR MIRIAM KINAI

ISBN: 1490522093

ISBN-13: 978-1490522098

CONTENTS

Acknowledgments   i

1   Diet Therapy   Pg #1

2   Supplements   Pg #5

3   Herbs   Pg #7

4   Aromatherapy   Pg #11

5   Lifestyle Modifications   Pg #25

ACKNOWLEDGMENTS

I would like to express my sincere gratitude to everyone who contributed in one way or another to the development of this publication.

I would especially like to thank http://www.zazzle.com/ChristianArtGifts for their photographs.

1

DIET THERAPY

Dietary modifications that you can institute to manage urinary tract infections naturally include:

1.

Drink Cranberry Juice

Studies have shown that drinking cranberry juice can clear as well as prevent UTI. It does this because of it contains proanthocyanins which stop the infection causing bacteria from adhering to the walls of the bladder, urethra and other parts of the urinary tract.

Therefore drink three glasses of pure cranberry juice every day if you have a UTI. Avoid the sweetened juices.

Do not take cranberry juice if you are taking blood thinners like warfarin since it may cause bleeding.

***

2.

Eat Blueberries

Blueberries can be eaten by themselves to clear UTIs. They can also be blended with cranberries to make a powerful UTI clearing cocktail.

***

3.

Drink Lots of Water

Drinking a lot of pure water can help clear a UTI and maintain a healthy urinary tract by flushing out the disease causing bacteria. Therefore drink half your weight in ounces of pure water every day. If you weigh 140 pounds drink 70 ounces of water.

***

4.

Eat Pineapples

Pineapples contain an enzyme called bromelain which has been shown to be help clear UTIs. They also contain other nutrients which strengthen the immune system and reduce inflammation like vitamin C. Therefore eat 1 cup of chopped pineapple each day if you have a UTI.

***

5.

Drink Baking Soda

Adding one tablespoon of baking soda to a glass of water and drinking the solution may help clear a UTI since it lowers the pH of the urine. This neutralizing of the acidic urine also helps reduce the painful burning sensation that is felt when urinating.

***

6.

Eat Vitamin C Rich Food

Eat foods which are rich in vitamin C since it boosts the immune system. Examples include oranges, grapefruits, tangerines, lemons and other citrus fruits.

***

7.

Take Apple Cider Vinegar

Apple cider vinegar is believed to help remove the UTI causing bacteria from the urinary tract.

***

8.

Eat Fermented Foods

Eating fermented foods like yogurt and cheese at least three times each week has been shown to reduce the frequency of getting UTIs in women.

Other fermented foods which are beneficial for the treatment of UTI since they increase the population of immune boosting good bacteria in your body include kefir, sauerkraut, kombucha made from milk.

***

9.

Eat Horseradish

Eating horseradish is also believed to be beneficial for the treatment of UTI since it has antibacterial properties.

***

10.

Reduce Alcohol Intake

Alcohol is thought to be a bladder irritant therefore reduce your consumption.

***

11.

Reduce Caffeine Intake

Caffeine is thought to be a bladder irritant therefore reduce your consumption of all coffee, caffeinated energy drinks and all other sources of caffeine.

***

12.

Reduce Sugar Intake

Sugar is thought to promote the growth of the UTI causing bacteria by reducing your body's ability to fight the infection. Therefore reduce your intake of soft drinks and sweeteners from cane sugar and corn syrup to agave syrup and honey.

* * * * *

2

SUPPLEMENTS

Nutritional supplements that can help manage UTIs include:

1.

Probiotics

Probiotics or healthy bacteria are useful for maintaining healthy urinary tracts. A good choice should contain 1 billion CFU (colon forming units) of Lactobacillus acidophilus and it can be taken thrice a day.

***

2.

D-Mannose

D-mannose is naturally found in cranberries and blueberries. It binds to UTI causing bacteria called E. coli and aids their being flushed out of the body. Mannose can be taken before sexual intercourse by those who are prone to having UTIs after sex. If you are trying to conceive, do not use D-Mannose since it can bind to sperm.

3.

Vitamin C

Vitamin C stimulates boosts the immune system by boosting levels of chemicals which block the multiplication of disease causing organisms. This anti-oxidant also acidifies the urine making it harder for the bacteria to flourish. A common dose is 1000 mg three times a day.

***

4.

Cranberry Extract

If you cannot tolerate the taste of unsweetened cranberry juice, take 400 mg of the cranberry extract each day.

***

5.

Garlic

Garlic is a natural immune booster and if you cannot tolerate the odor of fresh garlic, you can take garlic supplements.

***

6.

Daily Multivitamin

A multi-vitamin and multi-mineral supplement which contains the nutrients in their daily recommended values should be taken each day.

* * * * *

3

HERBS

Herbs that are used to manage UTIs include:

1.

Uva Ursi

Uva ursi (*Arctostaphylos uva-ursi*) has antiseptic properties which are useful for clearing the UTI causing bacteria.

Therefore take one cup of uva ursi tea per day and ensure that you also drink a lot of pure water. As you do so understand that it can turn your urine greenish brown.

Do not take uva ursi if you have kidney or liver disease or if you are pregnant or breastfeeding. Children should not be given uva ursi.

***

2.

Echinacea

Echinacea strengthens the immune system and has been used to treat UTIs.

***

3.

Peppermint

Peppermint contains menthols which kills bacteria. Therefore drink peppermint tea since it can be useful for helping clear UTI.

***

4.

Dandelion

Dandelion root tea mixed with nettle leaves is also used to treat UTIs.

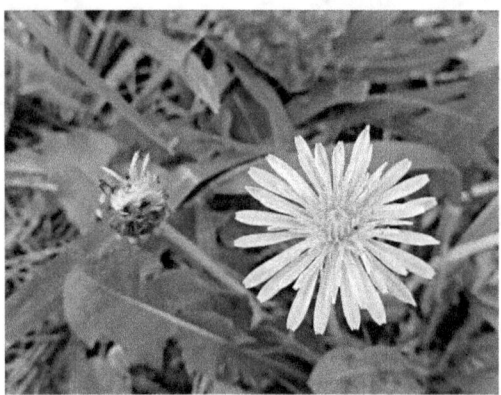

***

5.

Garlic

Garlic strengthens the immune system and helps fight infections by acting as a natural antibiotic.

Therefore, swallow the cloves raw or add them to your cooked dishes. You can also squeeze the garlic cloves and drink the fresh juice.

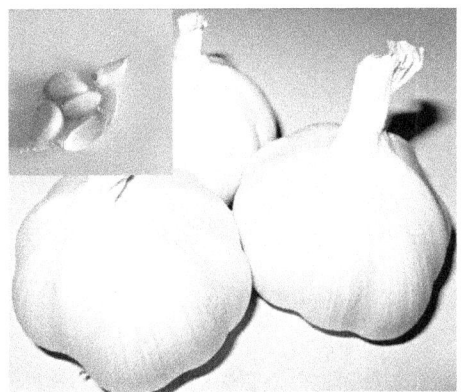

* * * * *

4

AROMATHERAPY

Aromatherapy is the use of essential oils for their healing benefits.

Aromatherapy oils which can be used to treat and prevent urinary tract infections include:

1. Essential oils with antiseptic (kills disease causing bacteria and viruses) properties like basil, bergamot, German chamomile, eucalyptus, frankincense, lavender, oregano, niaouli, palmarosa, pine, sandalwood, tea tree, thyme

2. Essential oils with diuretic (promotes the passing of urine) properties like cedarwood, cypress, fennel, juniper berry, pine, sandalwood, thyme

3. Essential oils with anti-inflammatory properties like bergamot, frankincense

4. Essential oils with immune boosting properties like tea tree, lavender, eucalyptus, bergamot

***

Bergamot Essential Oil

Botanical Name: Citrus bergamia

Method of Extraction: Expressed from fruit peel

Color: Yellowish green

Perfumery Note: Top note

Odor Intensity:

Strength of Initial Aroma: Medium

Aromatic Description: Citrusy and floral

**

Bergamot Essential Oil Safety Information

1. Do not expose the skin to sunlight and UV light for 12-24 hours after using it. It makes the skin more sensitive to the UV light and to developing skin cancer.

2. Do not use bergamot essential oil on children.

3. Do not use bergamot essential oil if you are pregnant or breastfeeding.

4. Avoid it if you have sensitive skin as it can irritate the skin.

5. Do not use bergamot if you are taking medications that make the skin more sensitive to sunlight. These include tetracycline, trimethoprim/sulfamethoxazole, amitriptyline, ciprofloxacin, levofloxacin and related drugs.

6. Do not use it alone for more than 2-3 months as it may lead to sensitization.

7. Always buy your essential oils from a reputable vender to ensure you use high quality therapeutic grade essential oils in your blends.

***

Eucalyptus Essential Oil

Botanical Name: Eucalyptus globulus

Method of Extraction: Steam distilled from the leaves

Color: Clear to yellow

Perfumery Note: Top note

Odor Intensity: 8

Strength of Initial Aroma: Strong

Aromatic Description: Fresh, camphoraceous, medicinal

Characteristics: Nontoxic, non-irritant and non-sensitizing.

**

Eucalyptus Essential Oil Safety Information

1. Do not ingest it as it can be fatal when taken orally.

2. Do not use it if you have epilepsy.

3. Do not use it if you have high blood pressure.

4. Do not apply it near a baby's nostrils.

5. Do not store it near homeopathic formulas as it may affect them.

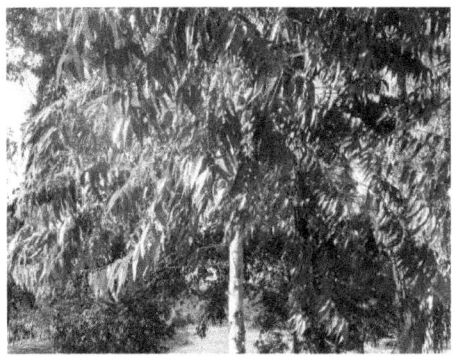

***

Lavender Essential Oil

Botanical Name: Lavendula officinalis

Method of Extraction: Steam distilled from the flowers

Color: Clear to yellow

Perfumery Note: Middle note

Odor Intensity: 4

Strength of Initial Aroma: Medium

Aromatic Description: Sweet, soothing, floral and fruity

Characteristics: Nontoxic, non-irritant and non-sensitizing. Can be used on all skin types

**

Lavender Essential Oil Safety Information

1. Do not use it in pregnancy especially the first 3 months.

2. Do not use it if you are breastfeeding.

3. Do not use it on young children as it may cause breast development in boys (gynaecomastia) and girls (pre-pubescent breast development).

4. Avoid it if you have low blood pressure as you may feel drowsy after using it.

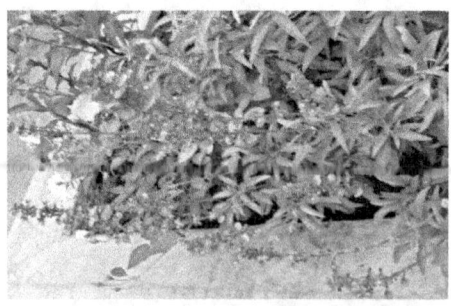

***

Sandalwood Essential Oil

Botanical Name: Santalum album

Method of Extraction: Steam distilled

Color: Clear to yellow

Perfumery Note: Base note

Odor Intensity: 5

Strength of Initial Aroma: Medium

Aromatic Description: Sweet, woody

Characteristics: Non-toxic, non-irritant, non-photo-toxic

**

Sandalwood Essential Oil Safety Information

1. Avoid using sandalwood if you are allergic to balsams.

2. Do not use it alone for more than 2-3 months as it may lead to sensitization.

3. Always buy your essential oils from a reputable vender to ensure you use high quality therapeutic grade essential oils in your blends.

4. Do not confuse essential oils with fragrance oils as the latter are not the natural essences.

***

Tea Tree Essential Oil

Botanical Name: Melaleuca alternifolia

Method of Extraction: Steam distilled

Color: Clear to yellow

Perfumery Note: Top note

Odor Intensity: 7

Strength of Initial Aroma: Strong

Aromatic Description: Fresh, medicinal, camphoraceous

**

Tea Tree Essential Oil Safety Information

1. It may be irritating on sensitive skins.

2. It may cause sweating when used in high concentrations. Maximum recommended level is 0.1%.

3. Do not use it alone for more than 2-3 months as it may lead to sensitization.

4. Always buy your essential oils from a reputable vender to ensure you use high quality therapeutic grade essential oils in your blends.

5. Do not confuse essential oils with fragrance oils as the latter are not the natural essences.

*****

Using Essential Oils for UTI Treatment

The first step in using essential oils to manage urinary tract infections is to do a patch test for each of the essential oils that you want to use.

To do this, simply apply the essential oil that has been diluted with a carrier oil on the inner aspect of your elbow, bandage it and wait for 24 hours to see if you will develop rashes or itchiness or swelling or any other sign of an allergic reaction. If you do, do not use that essential oil.

b) Add 2 drops of lavender essential oil, swirl and sniff

c) Add 3 drops of bergamot and 3 drops of tea tree eucalyptus essential oil, swirl and sniff

The second step is to create the essential oil blend that you will use to treat the UTI. A simple "UTI Blend" can be made by mixing 20 drops of lavender essential oil, 30 drops of bergamot essential oil, 30 drops of tea tree essential oil in a dark bottle.

We will refer to this mixture as "UTI Blend" in our recipes. Therefore, if the recipe says, "Add 12 drops of the UTI Blend", you simply add 12 drops of this mixture.

If you just want to buy one aromatherapy oil to experiment with, I would recommend tea tree essential oil. Likewise, if the recipe says, "Add 12 drops of the UTI Blend", you simply add 12 drops of tea tree essential oil.

Sitz Bath or Hip Bath.

Add 7 drops of the "UTI Blend" to water in a bowl that is large enough for you to sit in with the water reaching the hip level. Soak in it for 15 minutes. Repeat this twice or thrice a day.

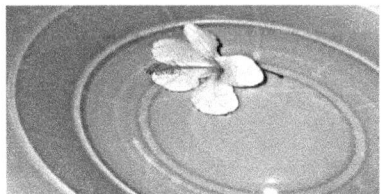

Aromatherapy Bath.

Create a healing bath by dispersing 20 drops of the "UTI Blend" in your warm bath water. You can also mix it with milk to help it disperse.

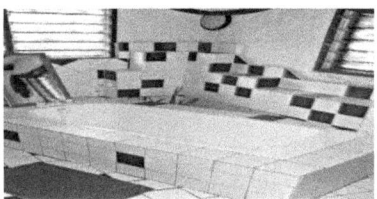

Bath Gel.

Add 50 drops (2.5 ml or ½ teaspoons) of the "UTI Blend" to one cup (8 oz or 250 ml) of unscented bath gel or liquid soap to create a healing bath gel.

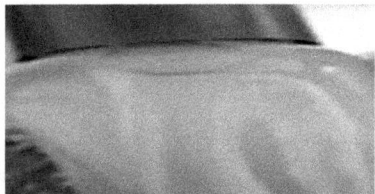

Body Massage Oil.

Add 50 drops (2.5 ml or ½ teaspoons) of the "UTI Blend" to one cup (8 oz or 250 ml) of sweet almond oil or any other carrier oil to create a UTI Treatment Body Massage Oil. Use it to massage your lower abdomen and back.

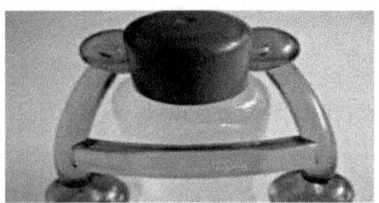

Abdominal Compress.

Add 25 drops (1.25 ml) of the "UTI Blend" to ½ cup (4 oz or 125 ml) of warm water and mix it, dip a hand towel in it and wring out the excess water. Apply it to your lower abdomen and rest for a few minutes as the healing oils penetrate. Once the towel cools, dip it in the warm water and repeat the process two or three times preferably after massaging the area with the UTI Treatment Body Massage Oil.

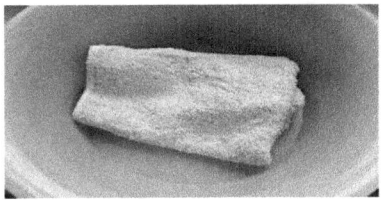

Body Wrap.

Add 20 drops of the "UTI Blend" to 3 oz or 100 ml of distilled water and spray it on a towel. Wrap your lower abdomen and back with the towel and then wrap a plastic sheet around yourself and relax for 20 minutes to give the healing oils time to penetrate before unwrapping yourself.

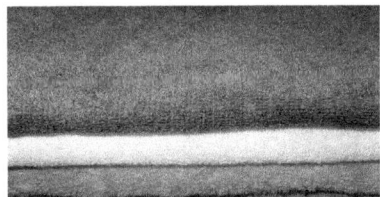

Back Compress.

Add 25 drops (1.25 ml or ¼ teaspoon) of the "UTI Blend" to ½ cup (4 oz or 125 ml) of warm water and mix it, dip a hand towel in it and wring out the excess water. Apply it to your back and rest for a few minutes as the healing oils penetrate. Once the towel cools, dip it in the warm water and repeat the process two or three times preferably after massaging the area with the UTI Treatment Body Massage Oil.

Body Oil.

Add 50 drops (2.5 ml or ½ teaspoons) of an immune boosting essential oil like tea tree, lavender, eucalyptus or bergamot essential oil to one cup (8 oz or 250 ml) of sweet almond oil or any other carrier oil to create a healing. Apply it to your skin after bathing and patting it dry but while it is still moist to lock in the moisture and healing benefits of the essential oil. As you apply it, pay special attention to the pelvis area, back and thighs.

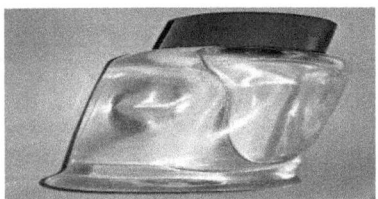

Panty Liner.

Add 6 drops of the "UTI Blend" to your panty liner or pad.

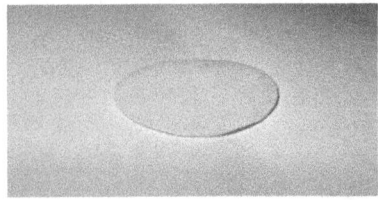

Aloe Vera Aromatherapy Gel.

Add 50 drops of the "UTI Blend" to one cup (8 oz or 250 ml) of natural aloe vera gel to create a non-greasy, healing moisturizer.

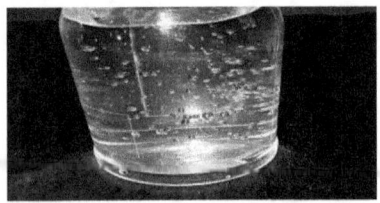

Healing Salve.

Melt 1 oz. (30 grams) of beeswax with 8 oz. (250 ml or 1 cup) of olive oil or any other vegetable oil in a double boiler. Remove from the heat source and one the mixture cools add up to 50 drops (2.5 ml or ½ teaspoon) of the "UTI Blend". Pour the mixture into storage tins and allow it to cool completely. Apply it to your lower abdomen and back.

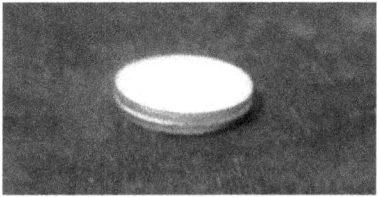

Body Lotion.

Heat 6 oz (190 ml) of sweet almond oil and 1.5 oz (45 grams) of grated beeswax in a double boiler until they mix. Remove from the heat and let the mixture cool completely. Put 8 oz (250 ml) water in a blender and with the blender on high speed, slowly pour in the cooled vegetable oil and beeswax mixture. Blend until the mixture emulsifies or forms a thick lotion. Add 10-20 drops of the "UTI Blend". Pour the lotion in a jar.

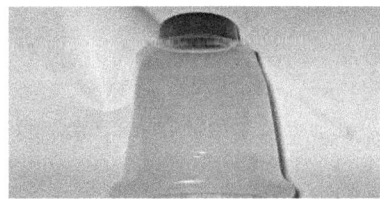

Healing Petroleum Jelly.

Melt 2 teaspoons of a petroleum jelly like Vaseline, add 6 drops of the "UTI Blend" when cool and then pour into a jar.

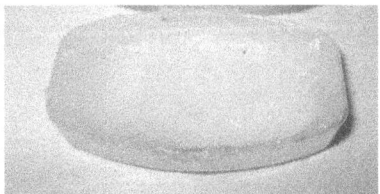

Facial Steamer.

Add 50 drops of an immune boosting essential oil like tea tree, lavender, eucalyptus or bergamot essential oil (or the number or drops recommended by the manufacturer) to one cup (8oz or 250 ml) of water and put it on your facial steamer or sauna.

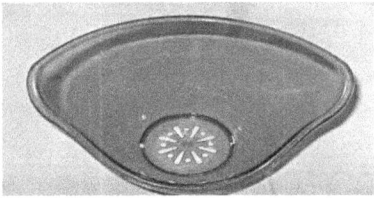

Scent Balls.

Add 6 drops of an immune boosting essential oil like tea tree, lavender, eucalyptus or bergamot essential oil to your handkerchief or a cotton ball and sniff it throughout the day.

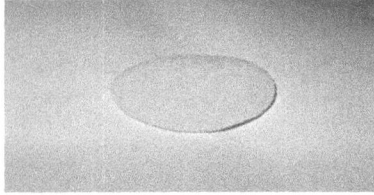

Scented Salts.

Mix 1 cup Epsom salts with 1 cup sea salt and add 50 drops (2.5 ml) of an immune boosting essential oil like tea tree, lavender, eucalyptus or bergamot essential oil in a glass jar with a tight lid. Open the jar and take a whiff of the scent several times during the day.

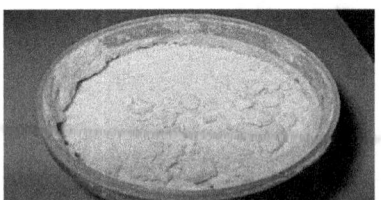

Room Fragrance.

Add 24 drops of an immune boosting essential oil like tea tree, lavender, eucalyptus or bergamot essential oil your diffuser. If your diffuser comes with instructions, use the number of drops recommended by the manufacturer.

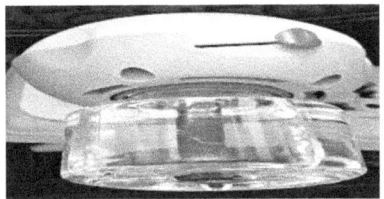

Room Scent.

Add 12 drops of an immune boosting essential oil like tea tree, lavender, eucalyptus or bergamot essential oil ¼ cup (2 oz or 60 ml) of water, place it on an oil warmer and light the candle to scatter the soothing scent.

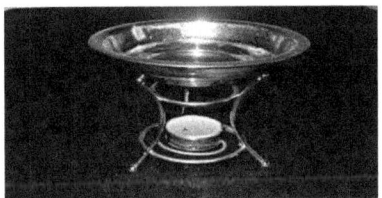

Air Freshener.

Create your own air freshener by adding a total of 250 drops (12.5 ml or 2.5 teaspoons) of an immune boosting essential oil like tea tree, lavender, eucalyptus or bergamot essential oil to one cup (8 oz or 250 ml) of water in a spray bottle and spray it around your room.

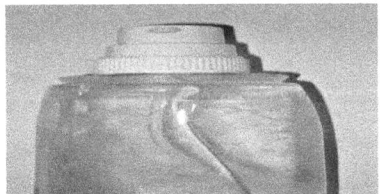

Light Bulb Scent.

Drop 3 drops of an immune boosting essential oil like tea tree, lavender, eucalyptus or bergamot essential oil to a light bulb when the light is switched off, switch it on to illuminate and scent your room.

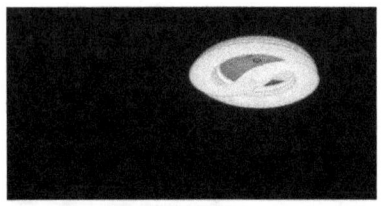

Aroma Ring Scent.

Add 5 drops of an immune boosting essential oil like tea tree, lavender, eucalyptus or bergamot essential oil to an aroma oil ring, place it on top of your lamp bulb, light the lamp and experience relaxing light.

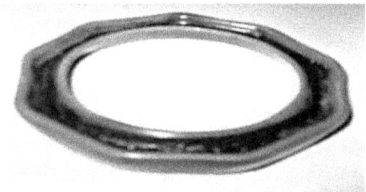

Car Diffuser.

Add an immune boosting essential oil like tea tree, lavender, eucalyptus or bergamot essential oil to your car's diffuser according to the manufacturer's instructions and let the healing scent envelope you as you drive.

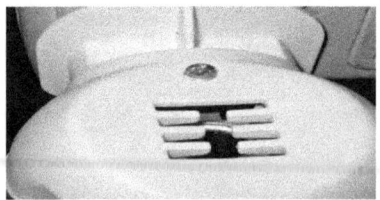

* * * * *

5

LIFESTYLE MODIFICATIONS

Lifestyle modifications that can help manage UTIs include:

1.

Do Not Hold Urine

Make it a habit to urinate whenever you feel the urge because holding urine helps the UTI causing bacteria multiply.

***

2.

Wipe From Front To Back

After using the toilet, wipe yourself from the front to the back so that you do not introduce bacteria into your urethra.

3.

Use White Unscented Toilet Paper

Avoid colored and scented toilet paper to prevent developing any reactions to dyes or perfumes in your genital area since this may make them more prone to becoming infected.

***

4.

Shower Instead Of Bathing

Take showers instead of long soaks in bath tubs and avoid Jacuzzis and hot tubs.

***

5.

Clean Up Before Sex

Clean your genital area before sexual intercourse because this reduces the population of bacteria and thereby reduces their chances of gaining access into your urethra. You can take a full bath or simply use flushable wipes.

***

6.

Use Gentle Cleansers

Avoid using scented soaps and bath gels and clean the genital area with gentle cleansers to avoid irritating the delicate tissues.

***

7.

Urinate After Sex

Urinate after sex to get rid of any bacteria in your bladder so that they do not multiply and cause or worsen an existing infection.

***

8.

Avoid Feminine Hygiene Sprays

Avoid using feminine hygiene sprays and douches since they can dry or irritate the delicate tissues of the urethra and vagina and thus make it easier for infections to develop.

***

9.

Wear Cotton Underwear

Wear white, loose cotton underwear or undergarments with cotton crotches to keep the genital area dry since cotton absorbs the moisture.

###

ABOUT THE AUTHOR

Dr. Miriam Kinai is a medical doctor and a certified clinical aromatherapy practitioner.

You can visit her blog at http://www.MyBlogBookClub.com or follow her on twitter at http://twitter.com/AlmasiHealth

Email enquiries to almasihealthcare@yahoo.com with BOOKS as your subject.

HERBS AND SPICES FOR THE COOK, HEALER AND BEAUTICIAN

Herbs and Spices for the Cook, Healer and Beautician uses color pictures and clear explanations to teach you about more than 70 healing herbs and spices.

You will learn about their:

* Therapeutic (healing) uses

* Drug interactions

* Contraindications (when not to use them)

* Cooking tips

* Beauty tips

*****

INTERNATIONAL GOURMET HERB AND SPICE BLENDS

International Gourmet Herb and Spice Blends teaches you how to prepare exotic herb and spice blends from around the world. You will discover the recipes for:

* Barbecue Rub, Cajun, Apple Pie and Pumpkin Pie Spice Mixes from America

* Pudding Spice Mix from Britain

* 5 Spice Mix from China

* Berbere Spice Mix from Ethiopia

* Curry Powder and Garam Masala from India

* Bouquet Garni, Herbs de Provence and Quatre Epices from France

* Herb Mix from Italy

* Jerk Seasoning from Jamaica

* Shichimi Togarashi from Japan

* Pilau Spice Blend from Kenya

* Chili Powder from Mexico

* Baharat Spice Blend from the Middle East

* Ras El Hanout from Morocco

*****

THE QUICK GOURMET CHEF

The Quick Gourmet is an essential culinary skills cookbook which teaches how to make simple, divine dishes.

You will learn how to make:

* Hot Chocolate Mixes and Drinks

* Hot Chai Tea Mixes and Drinks

* Hot Coffee Mixes and Drinks

* Sensational Smoothies

* Non-Dairy Smoothies

* Chocolate Covered Strawberries

* Chocolate Truffles

* Healthy Chicken Salads

* Healthy Tuna Salads

* Savory Salsas

* Herb Butter

* Cheese Dips and Sauces

* Gourmet Sandwiches

* Perfect Hard Boiled Eggs

* A Cheese Board

* Natural Food Color

*****

HOW TO STYLE AND PHOTOGRAPH FOOD

Regardless of whether you are an aspiring food blogger or you want to make money online selling stock photos, How To Style and Photograph Food, uses color pictures and clear explanations to teach you the food photography tips that can help you improve your digital camera photography skills so that you can begin photographing food like a pro.

You will learn:

* The equipment that you need

* How to set up the lighting

* How to prepare the stage

* How to style the food

* How to shoot the food

*****

HOW TO MAKE NATURAL SKIN CARE PRODUCTS VOLUME 1

How To Make Natural Skin Care Products Volume 1 by Dr Miriam Kinai is filled with recipes for making organic bath and body products for normal, sensitive, oily and dry skin types as well as therapeutic products to manage mature skin, prematurely aging skin, cellulite, eczema, psoriasis, ringworms, dandruff, thinning hair, menopausal symptoms, pre-menstrual tension (PMS), painful periods, arthritis, stress, sadness or depression, mental exhaustion and insomnia.

This book also teaches you the best vegetable oils, essential oils, natural butters and herbs to use when making products for different skin types physical conditions. You will learn how to make:

* Bath bombs

* Bath melts

* Bath salts

* Bath teas

* Body butters

* Body lotions

* Body scrubs

* Healing balms and body creams

* Herb infused oils

* Natural soap

How to Make Natural Skin Care Products Volume 1 will leave you with a clear understanding of how to make bath and beauty products to use in your home or to give as gifts or to sell and make money.

*****

ORGANIC SKIN CARE PRODUCT INGREDIENTS

Organic Skin Care Product Ingredients teaches you about the different natural substances that can be used to create natural bath and beauty products to use in your home or to give as gifts to your loved ones or to sell and make money.

You will learn about:

* Natural butters

* Natural clays

* Natural colorants

* Natural exfoliants

* Natural fragrances

* Natural oils

* Natural preservatives

*****

THE ESSENTIALS OF AROMATHERAPY ESSENTIAL OILS

The Essentials of Aromatherapy Essential Oils by Dr Miriam Kinai teaches you how to use aromatherapy oils to improve your physical, mental and emotional well being.

The author's experience as a medical doctor and clinical aromatherapy practitioner have enabled her to write a highly informative guide for those who want to utilize the healing benefits of these natural plant essences.

You will discover:

* The safety information and therapeutic uses of 18 essential oils

* How to blend essential oils

* The characteristics and uses of 14 carrier oils

* How to Dilute Essential Oils with Carrier Oils

* How to Use Essential Oils

* Cautionary Measures when using Essential Oils

* Numerous Essential Oil Recipes for bath products as well as skin care and hair care products

The Essentials of Aromatherapy Essential Oils will leave you with a clear understanding of how you can safely use aromatherapy essential oils to heal yourself naturally.

*****

CARRIER OILS GUIDE

Carrier Oils Guide teaches you the characteristics, health benefits and uses of commonly used carrier oils. You will learn about:

* Apricot Kernel Oil

* Avocado Oil

* Borage Seed Oil

* Calendula Oil

* Carrot Seed Oil

* Castor Oil

* Evening Primrose Oil

* Fractionated Coconut Oil

* Jojoba

* Olive Oil

* Rosehip Oil

* Sunflower Oil

* Sweet Almond Oil

* Virgin Coconut Oil

* Useful formulas for Diluting Essential Oils with Carrier Oils

*****

MEDICAL AROMATHERAPY FOR HEALTH PROFESSIONALS

Medical Aromatherapy for Healthcare Professionals by Dr Miriam Kinai teaches you how to use essential oils to treat physical diseases and emotional disorders.

The author's experience as a medical doctor and clinical aromatherapy practitioner have enabled her to write a highly informative guide for those who want to utilize the healing benefits of these natural plant essences.

You will discover how to use essential oils to:

* Treat skin diseases like acne, eczema and psoriasis

* Treat other physical diseases like high blood pressure, arthritis, coughs and colds

* Manage mental and emotional conditions like anxiety, depression, anger and stress

* Relieve the symptoms of menopause and premenstrual tension

* Lessen insomnia and impotence

Medical Aromatherapy for Healthcare Professionals is therefore an essential resource for holistic healthcare practitioners like massage therapists, naturopaths and herbalists.

It is also a useful resource for conventional medicine healthcare providers like physicians and nurses who want to begin practicing integrative medicine and for patients who want to improve their health naturally by using aromatherapy oils.

*****

AROMATHERAPY COURSE

Aromatherapy Course by Dr Miriam Kinai tutors you on how to use essential oils to improve your physical, mental and emotional well being.

The author's experience as a medical doctor and clinical aromatherapy practitioner have enabled her to create a highly informative course on how to use these natural plant essences.

You will learn:

* The safety information and therapeutic uses of essential oils like clary sage, eucalyptus, geranium, grapefruit, lavender, lemon, lemongrass, marjoram, orange (sweet), patchouli, peppermint, Roman chamomile, rose, rosemary, sandalwood, spearmint, tea tree and ylang ylang.

* The safety information and therapeutic uses of carrier oils like apricot kernel oil, avocado oil, borage seed oil, calendula oil, carrot seed oil, castor oil, evening primrose oil, fractionated coconut oil, jojoba, olive oil, rosehip oil, sunflower oil, sweet almond oil and virgin coconut oil.

* How to blend essential oils

* How to dilute essential oils with carrier oils

* How to administer essential oils

* How to make natural healing products from numerous aromatherapy recipes

* How to utilize the healing benefits of essentials oils even if you do not have prior training in aromatherapy

The Aromatherapy Course will leave you with a clear understanding of how you can heal yourself and your family naturally by using essentials oils on your body and in your home.

*****

DEALING WITH DEPRESSION NATURALLY

Dealing with Depression Naturally presents a holistic approach to managing depression with natural antidepressants. You will learn how to treat depression with:

* Aromatherapy

* Art therapy

* Christian Biblical principles

* Chromotherapy

* Diet therapy

* Eco-therapy

* Herbal therapy

* Home decor therapy

* Music therapy

* Phototherapy

* Exercise therapy

* Self-Psychotherapy

* Social therapy

* Talk therapy

* Vitamin therapy

* Writing therapy

*****

CHRISTIAN LIFE COACHING HANDBOOK

Christian Life Coaching Handbook offers a Biblical approach to managing different aspects of life.

You will learn:

* Christian anger management

* Christian conflict resolution

* Christian depression treatment

* Christian goal setting

* Christian marital stress management

* Christian stress management

* How to assert yourself

* How to defeat fear

* How to love yourself

* How to overcome shyness

* How to resist temptation

* How to stop being a people pleaser

*****

CHRISTIAN PERSONAL FINANCE

Christian Personal Finance teaches Biblical principles of money management.

You will learn:

* Christian financial stress management from people who were dealing with money stress like the Acts 3 beggar or credit issues like the widow in second Kings.

* Biblical prosperity principles from wealthy men and women of God like Isaac and the Proverbs 31 woman.

* Bible verses to use as **spiritual warfare prayers** and as Christian finance affirmations and Christian money meditations.

*****

ANTHOLOGY OF CHRISTIAN BIBLE SERMONS

Anthology of Christian Bible Sermons is a compilation of more than 20 Biblical rhema teachings which include:

* A New Christmas Message

* A New Easter Message

* Are You A Flamboyant Fig Tree Christian?

* Biblical Lessons for Purim from Queen Esther

* Can God Help Me If I Am Surrounded By Enemies?

* How Badly Do You Really Want It?

* Seed Words And The Powerful Tongue

* Spiritual AIDS

* The Three Levels Of Getting Lost

* Why Does God Allow Suffering?

* Your Life Is Your Ministry And Your Storm Is Your Message

* A Perfect God, Imperfect People, and Perfect Plans

* We Are Not Ignorant of His Devices

* How to Prepare for a Dangerous Journey

* Yes, God Can

* How to Serve the Body of Christ

* Conduits of God

* Go Back? Stand Still? Move Forward? Drown?

*****

CHRISTIAN SPIRITUAL WARFARE

Christian Spiritual Warfare teaches you the awesome Bible verses you can use as spiritual warfare prayers, Christian affirmations and in your Christian meditation sessions as you fight your spiritual battles.

You will learn how to fight for the following with Bible verses:

* Marriage * Children * Health

* Christian Faith * Christian Ministry

* Country

* Finances * Job * Business

* Peace of Mind * Restoration * Self Esteem * Self Love

You will also learn how to fight against the following with Bible verses:

* Addiction * Temptation

* Being Single * Infertility

* Opposition * Oppression

* Worry * Fear

* Feelings of Condemnation * Confusion

* Danger * Death * Despair * Discouragement

* Impatience * Insomnia * Laziness * Loneliness

* Poverty * Pride * Sadness

* Vengeance * Weakness

* A Foul Mouth * Lying

*****

DARK SKIN DERMATOLOGY COLOR ATLAS

Dark Skin Dermatology Color Atlas is filled with clear explanations and color photos of skin, hair, and nail diseases affecting people with skin of color or Fitzpatrick skin types IV, V, and VI.

Topics covered include Acne Vulgaris, Alopecia Areata, Anal Warts, Angioedema, Aphthous Ulcers, Atopic Dermatitis, Blastomycosis, Blister Beetle Dermatitis or Nairobi Fly Dermatitis, Cellulitis, Chronic Ulcers, Confetti Hypopigmentation, Cutaneous T Cell Lymphoma, Cutaneous Tuberculosis, Dermatitis Artefacta, Erythema Nodosum,

Exfoliative Erythroderma, Gianotti Crosti Syndrome, Hand Dermatitis, Hemangioma, Herpes Zoster, Ichthyosis, Ingrown Toenails, Irritant Contact Dermatitis, Kaposi Sarcoma, Keloids, Keratoderma Blenorrhagica, Klippel Trenaunay Weber Syndrome, Leishmaniasis, Leprosy, Leukonychia, Lichen Nitidus, Lichen Planus,

Lichenoid Drug Eruption, Linear Epidermal Nevus, Linear IgA Dermatosis (LAD), Lipodermatosclerosis, Lymphangioma Circumscriptum, Miliaria, Molluscum Contagiosum, Neurofibromatosis, Nickel Dermatitis, Onychomadesis, Onychomycosis, Palmoplantar Eccrine Hidradenitis, Papular Pruritic Eruption (PPE), Paronychia, Pellagra, Pemphigus Foliaceous,

Pemphigus Vulgaris, Piebaldism, Pityriasis Rosea, Pityriasis Rubra Pilaris, Plantar Hyperkeratosis, Plantar Warts, Poikiloderma, Postinflammatory Hyperpigmentation and Hypopigmentation, Post Topical Steroids Hypopigmentation, Psoriasis, Pyogenic Granuloma or Lobular Capillary Hemangioma, Scabies, Seborrheic Dermatitis, Steven Johnson Syndrome (SJS) and Toxic Epidermal Necrolysis (TEN),

Sunburn, Systemic Sclerosis, Tinea Capitis, Tinea Pedis, Tinea Versicolor, Traction Alopecia, Urticaria, Vasculitis, Vitiligo, and Xanthelasma.

*****